For the parents whose little ones keep them awake through the night:

Sometimes, all you can do is lie in bed, and hope
to fall asleep before you fall apart.
— William C. Hannan

And for the children, wide-awake, when all the birds are sleeping:

The sun has gone to bed and so must I.
— Oscar Hammerstein & Richard Rodgers

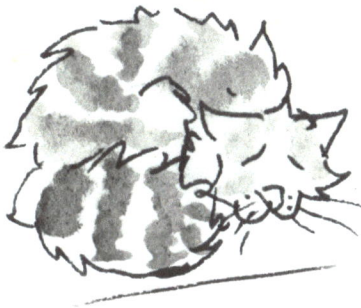

"My CPAP is OKAY"
Endorsed by:

David A. Walker, D.O., D.ABSM

Cindy Nichols, Ph.D., FAASM, CBSM, D.ABSM

Margaret Moen, M.D., ABSM, ABN

Zoe Anne Turner, CRT, PRGT, RST

Nancy Harris, RN, MSN, FNP-BC

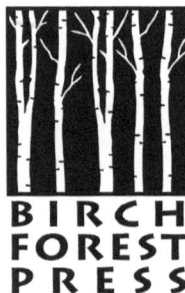

BIRCH FOREST PRESS

To order additional copies email for more information:
BirchForestPress@aye.net
www.BirchForestPress.com

My CPAP is Okay!

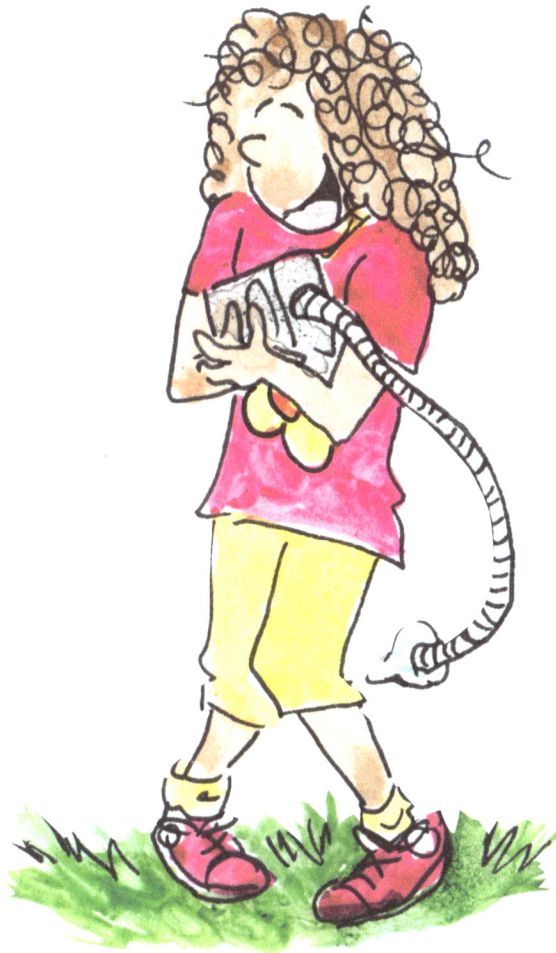

Barbara Disborough, MA, RRT

Artwork by Suzanne R. Sudekum

Hi!
My name is Stephie.
I am 5 years old.

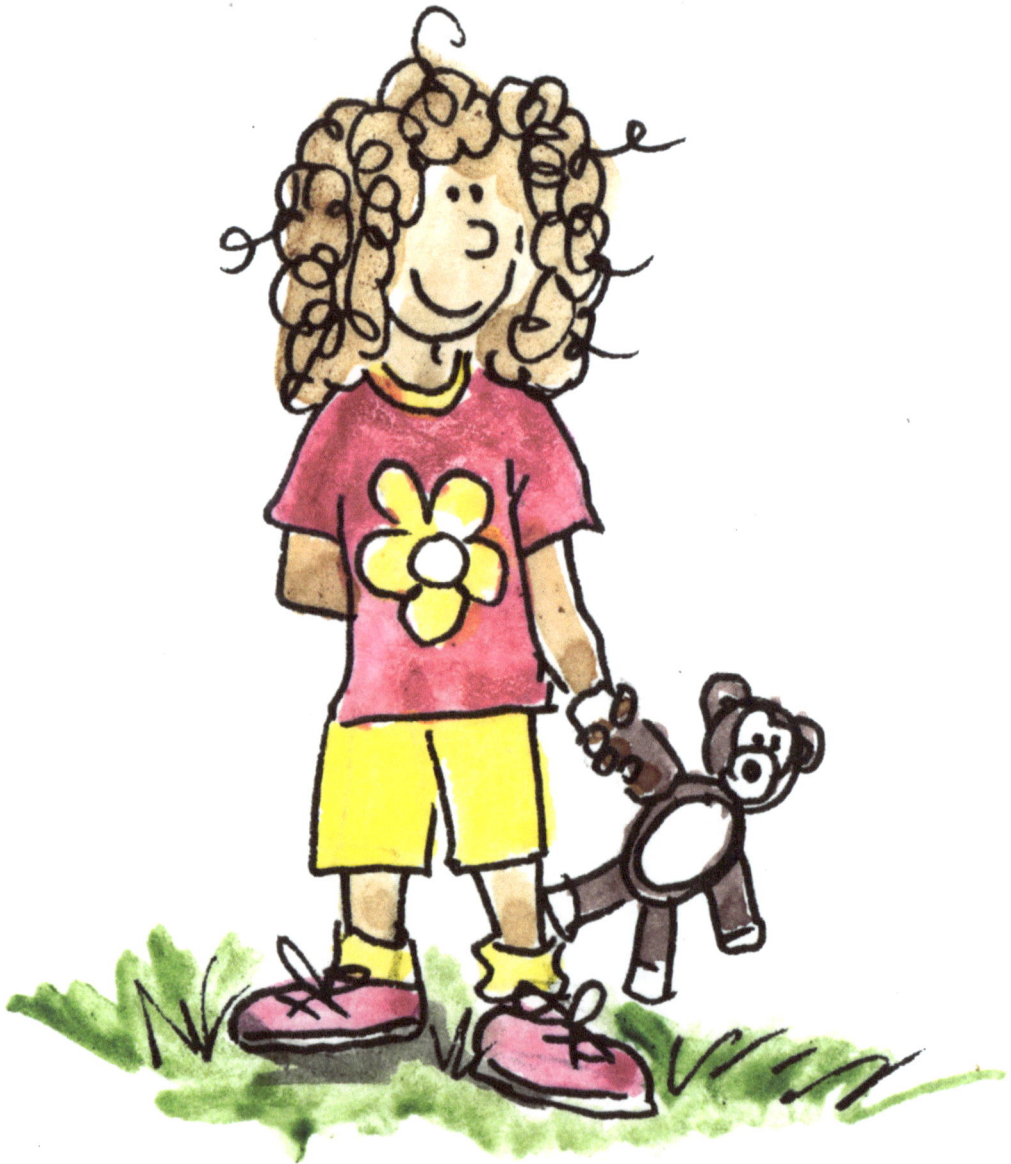

I live with my mom
and my dad.

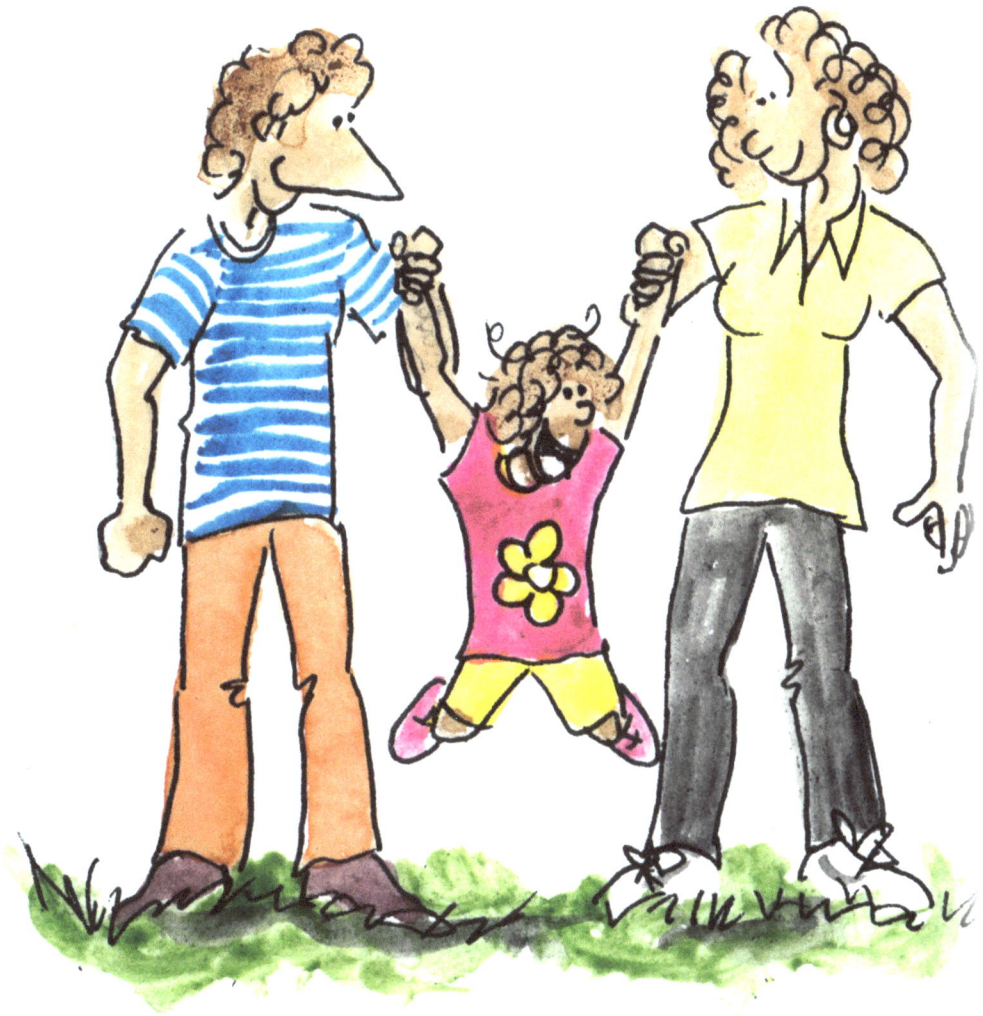

And my brother,
Danny.

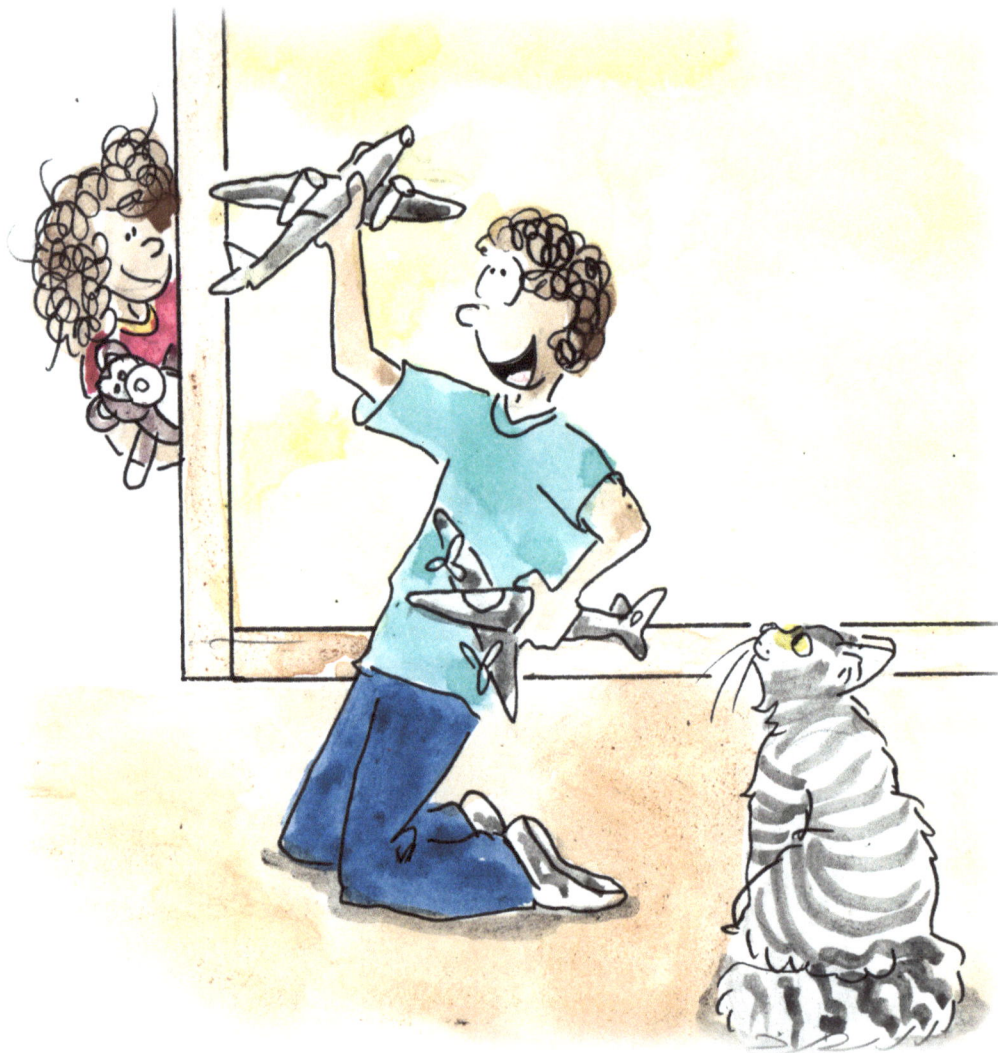

And my cat,
Gracie.

I go to pre-school and I
like to learn new things.

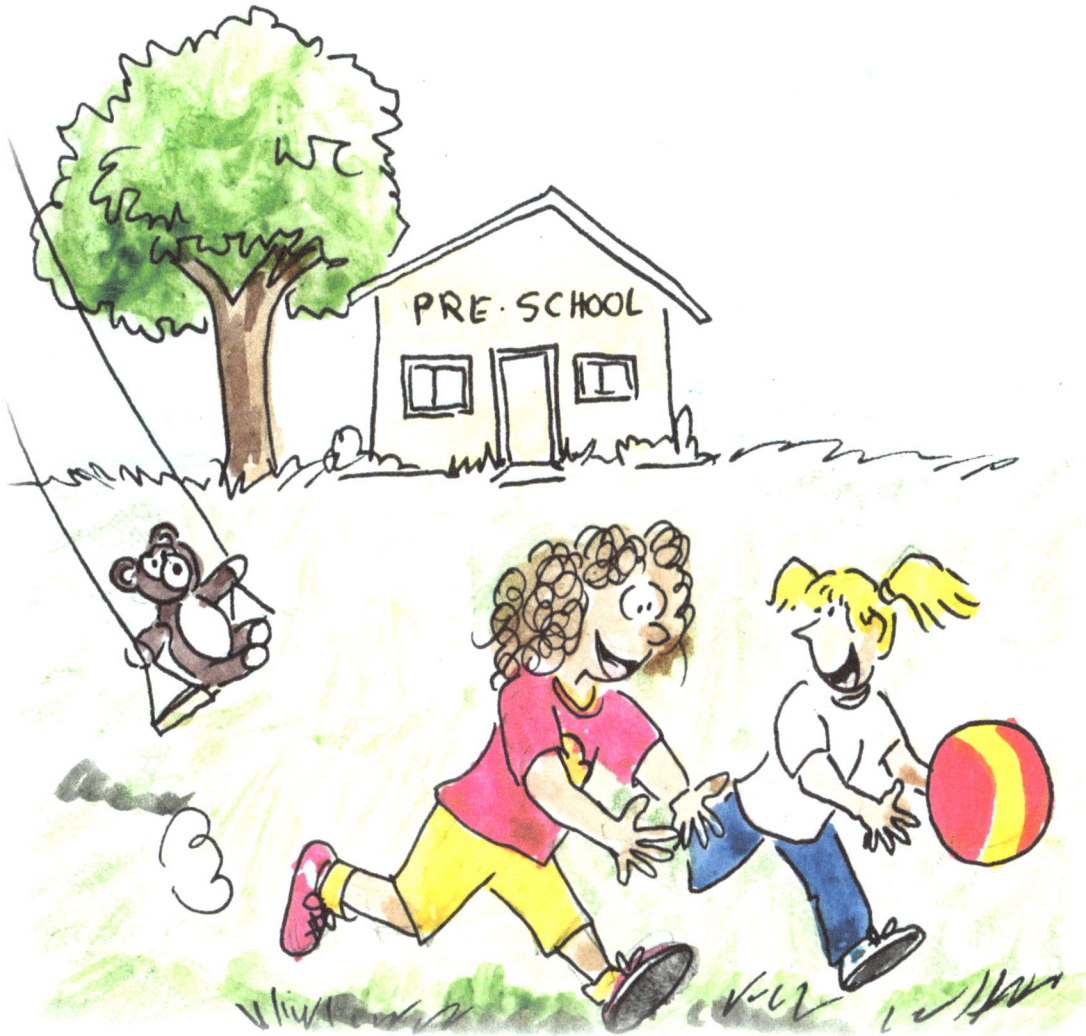

I have a lot of fun
playing with my friends.

My grandma says I am special. My Grandpa says everyone is special, but that I am EXTRA special.

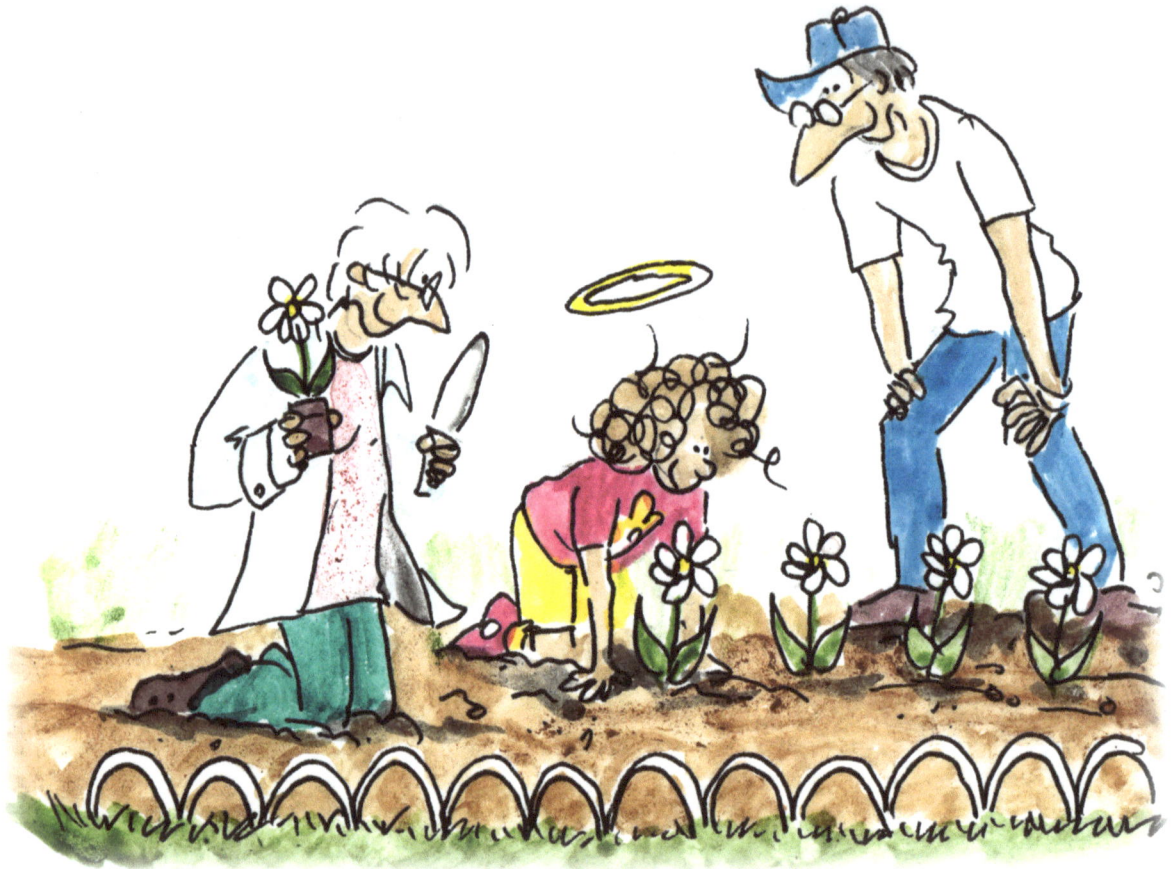

I asked him HOW I am special. I thought he would say I was his little angel.

He said it is because I have a special sleep machine.

Mom and dad think that I don't sleep very well.

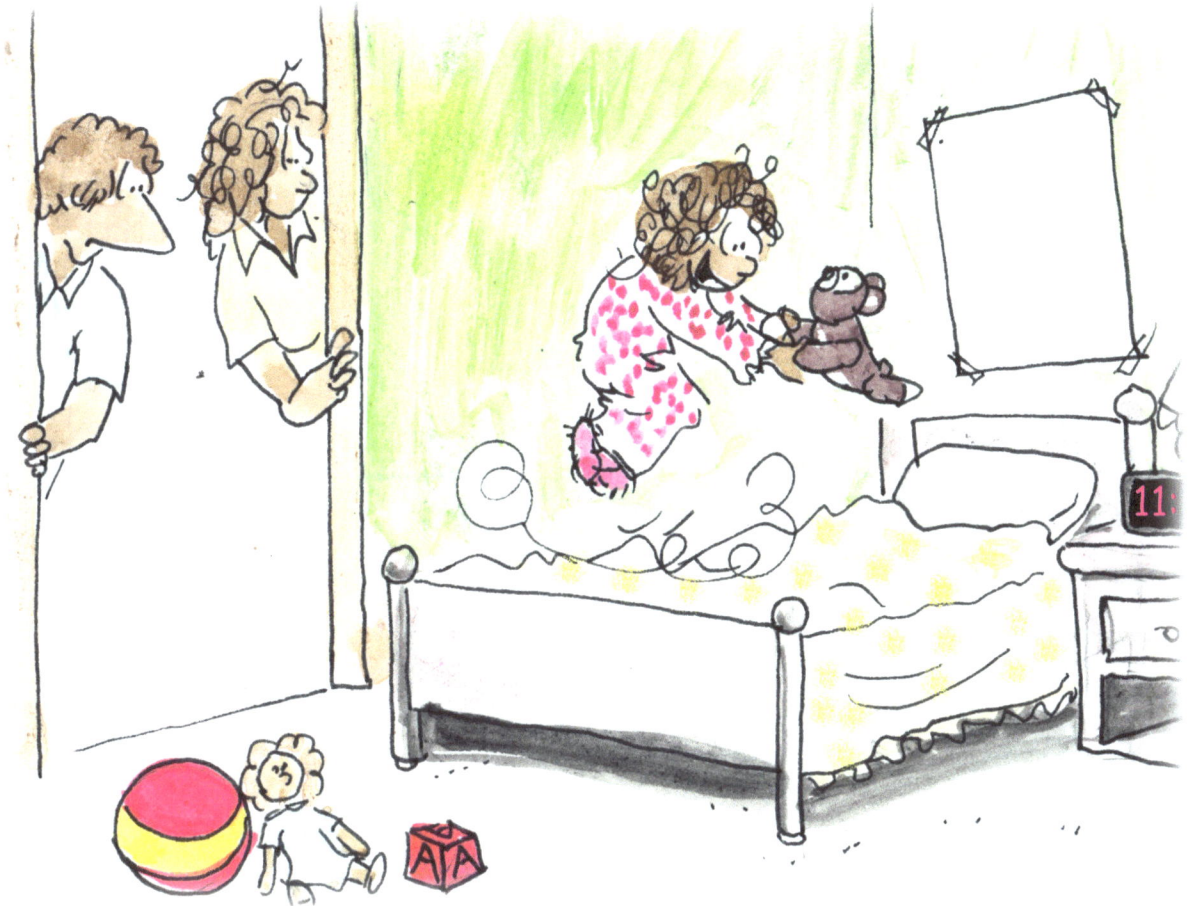

I think I sleep just FINE, thank you!

I also snore.
That's what THEY say.

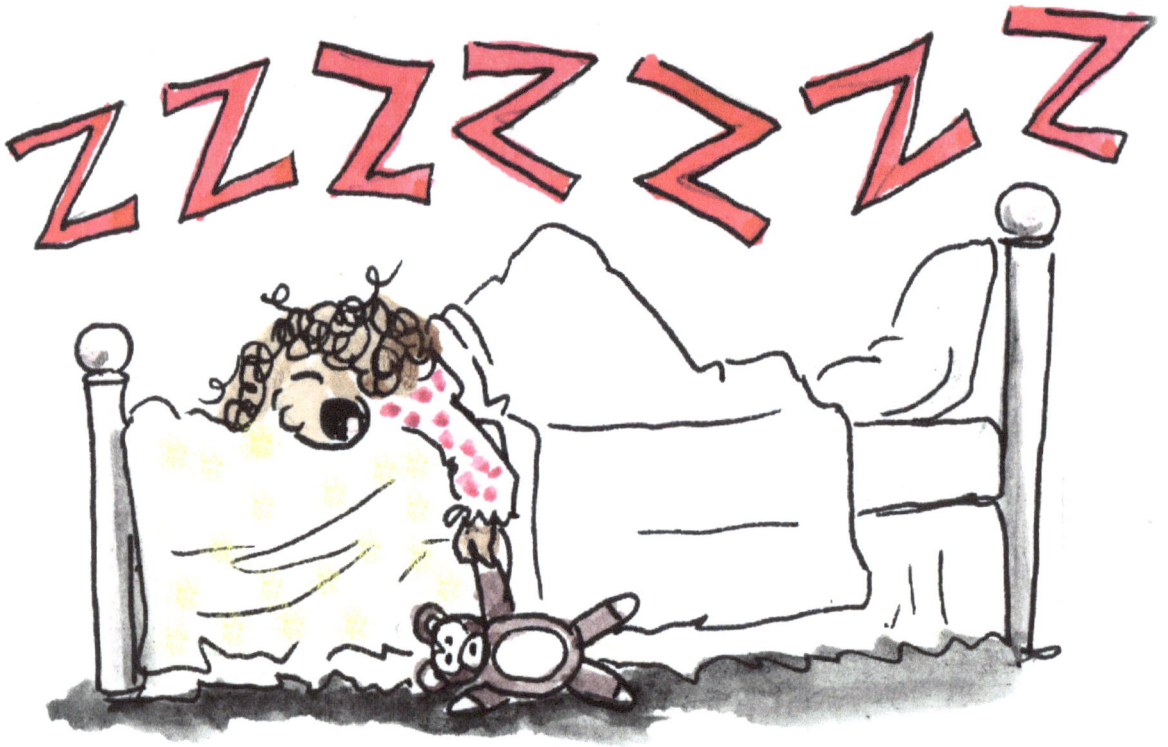

I AM sleeping so I don't know. So
I said "SO WHAT!!"

Mommy says I snore so loud she covers her ears.

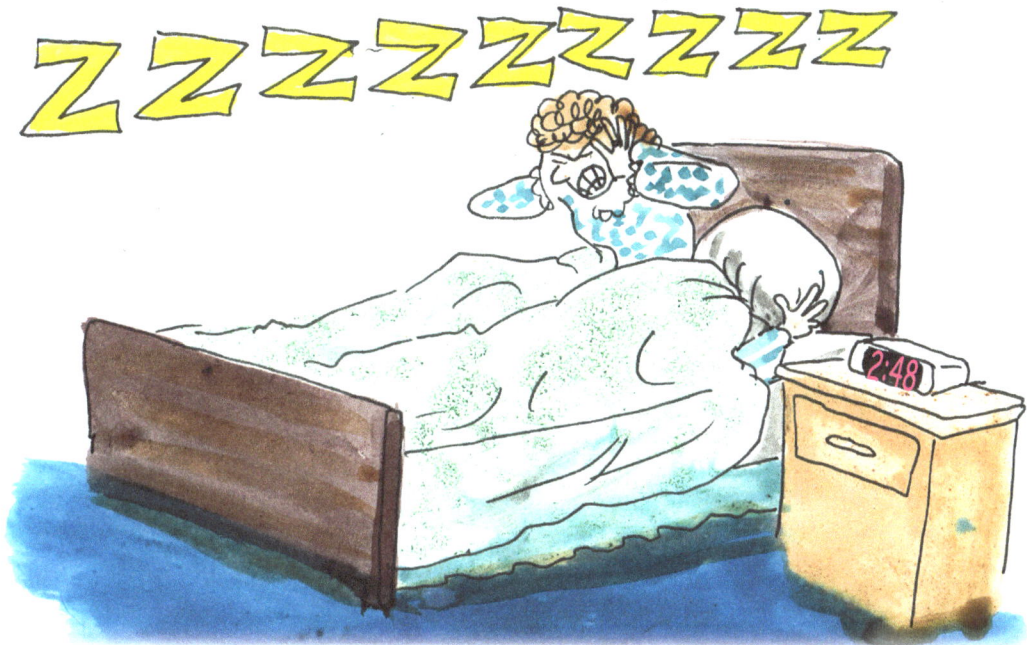

Danny says I snore so loud he thinks he's at the airport.

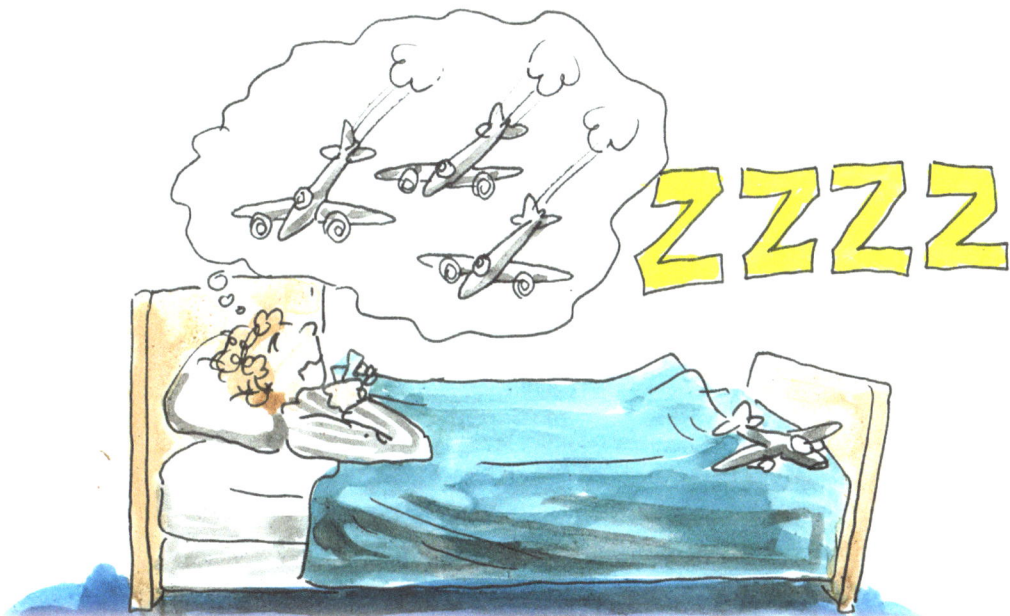

Daddy says I snore SO LOUD I make the house shake.

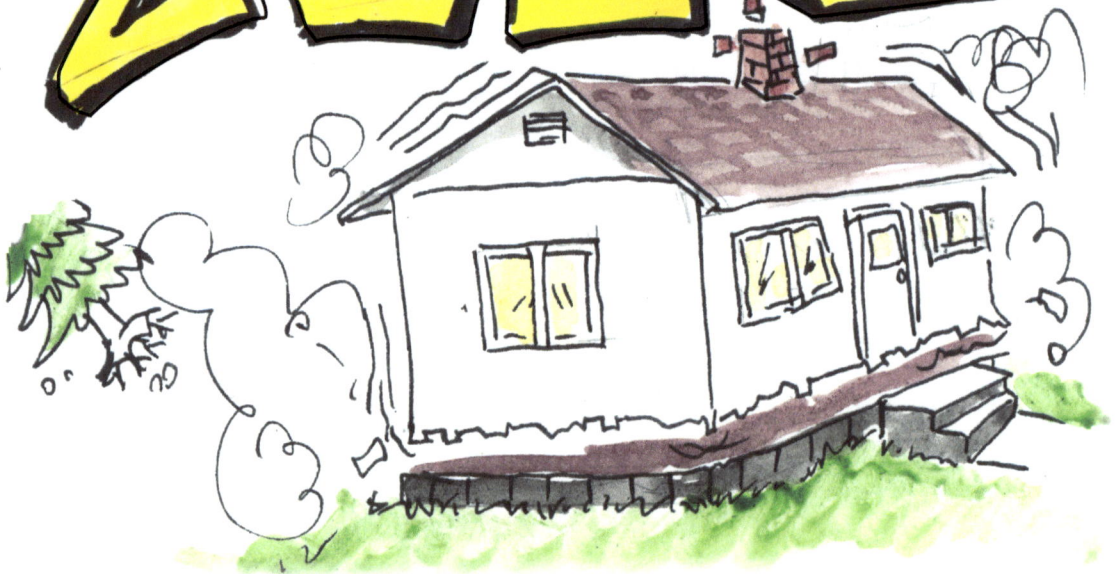

...OK, not really THAT loud.

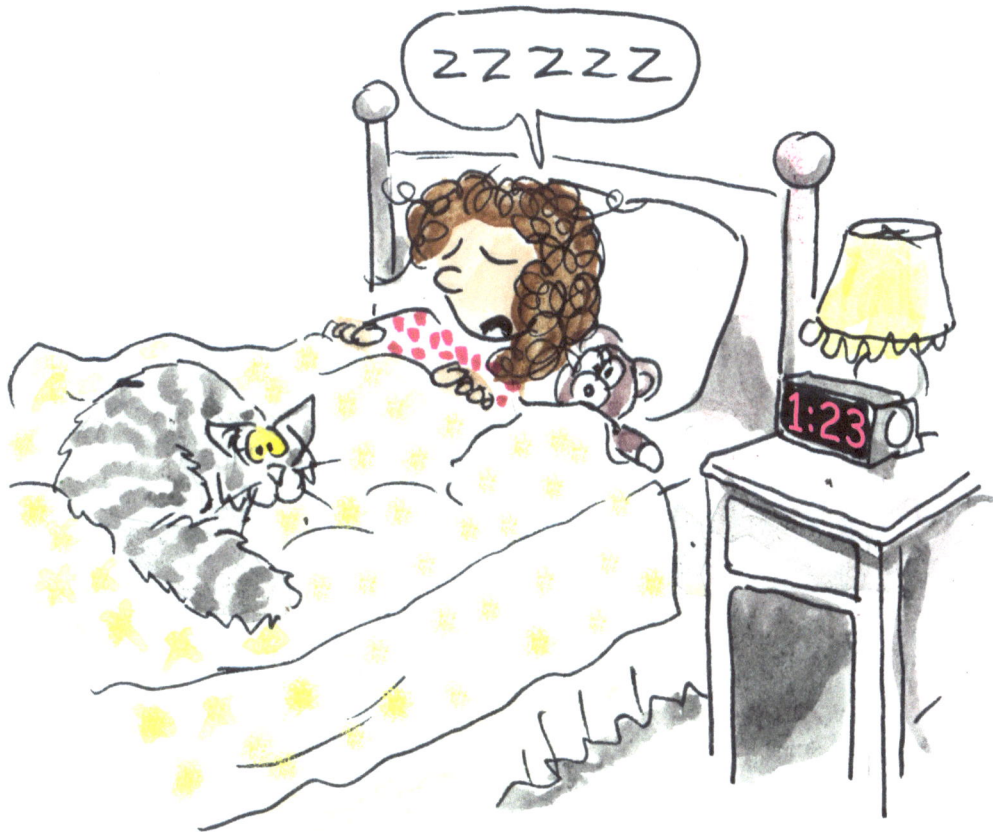

Once I went to a sleep-over for Sally's birthday. We stayed up and ate popcorn and played.

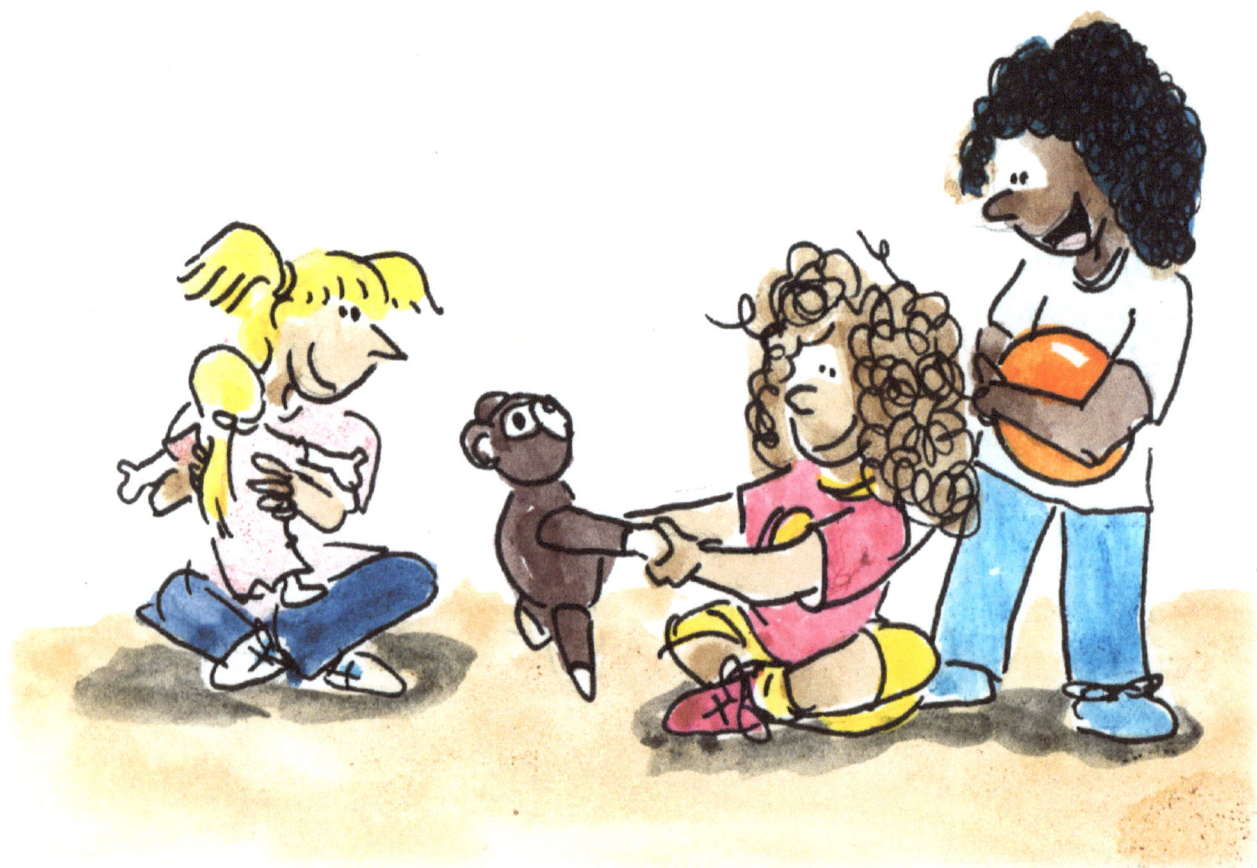

And then we all went to sleep in our sleeping bags.

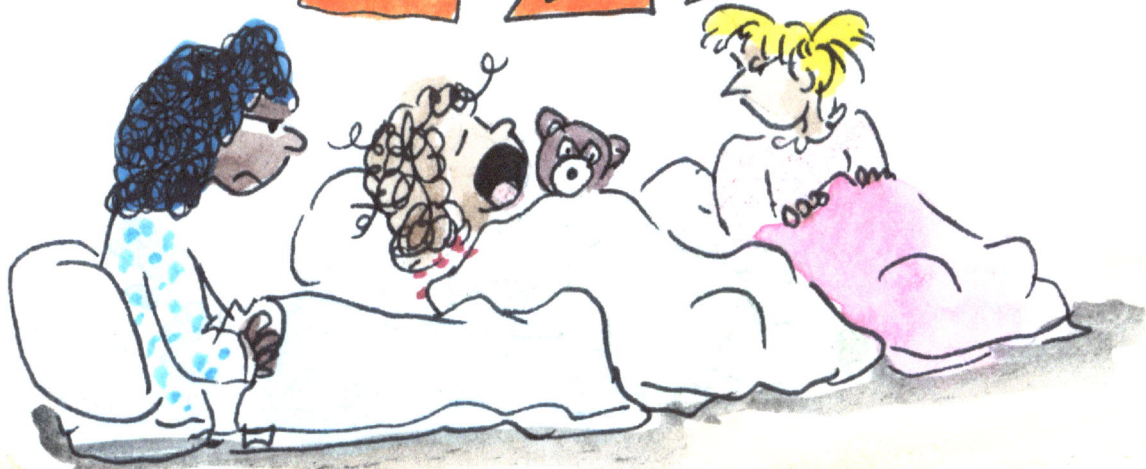

In the morning her dad fixed us breakfast.

Everyone was grumpy and tired, and they said I kept them awake all night.

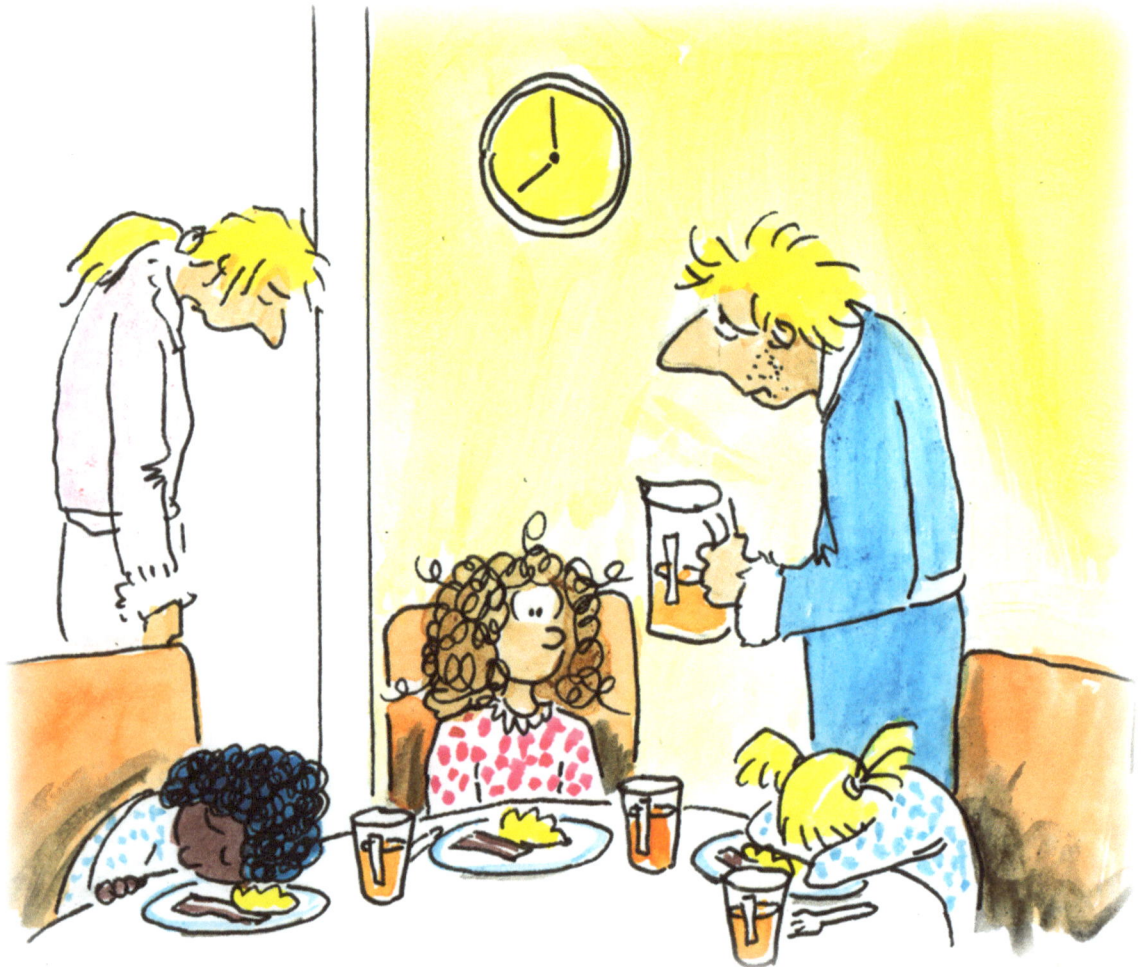

They told me I snored!

Last week I didn't get invited to a slumber party.

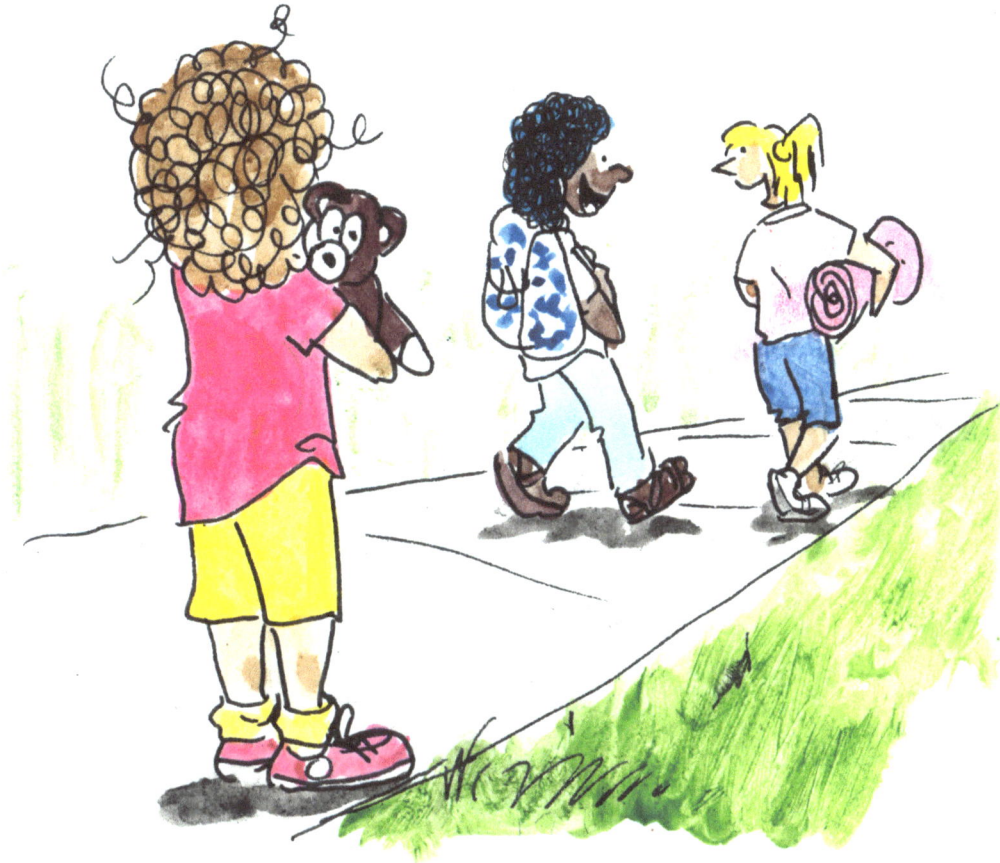

They said "maybe next time" and we all know what THAT means.

It means I'm not invited because I snored last time.

Sometimes I fall asleep
in school.

ZZZZZZ

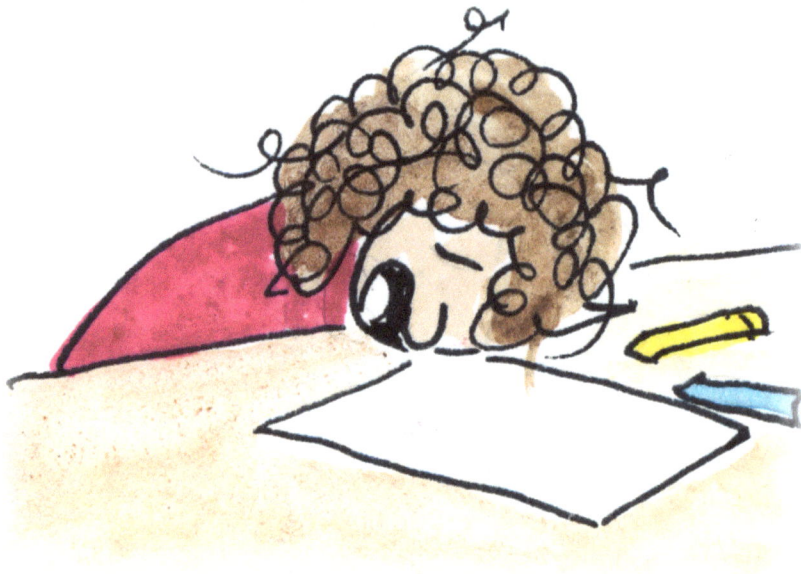

And dad says I am way too grumpy for a little girl...

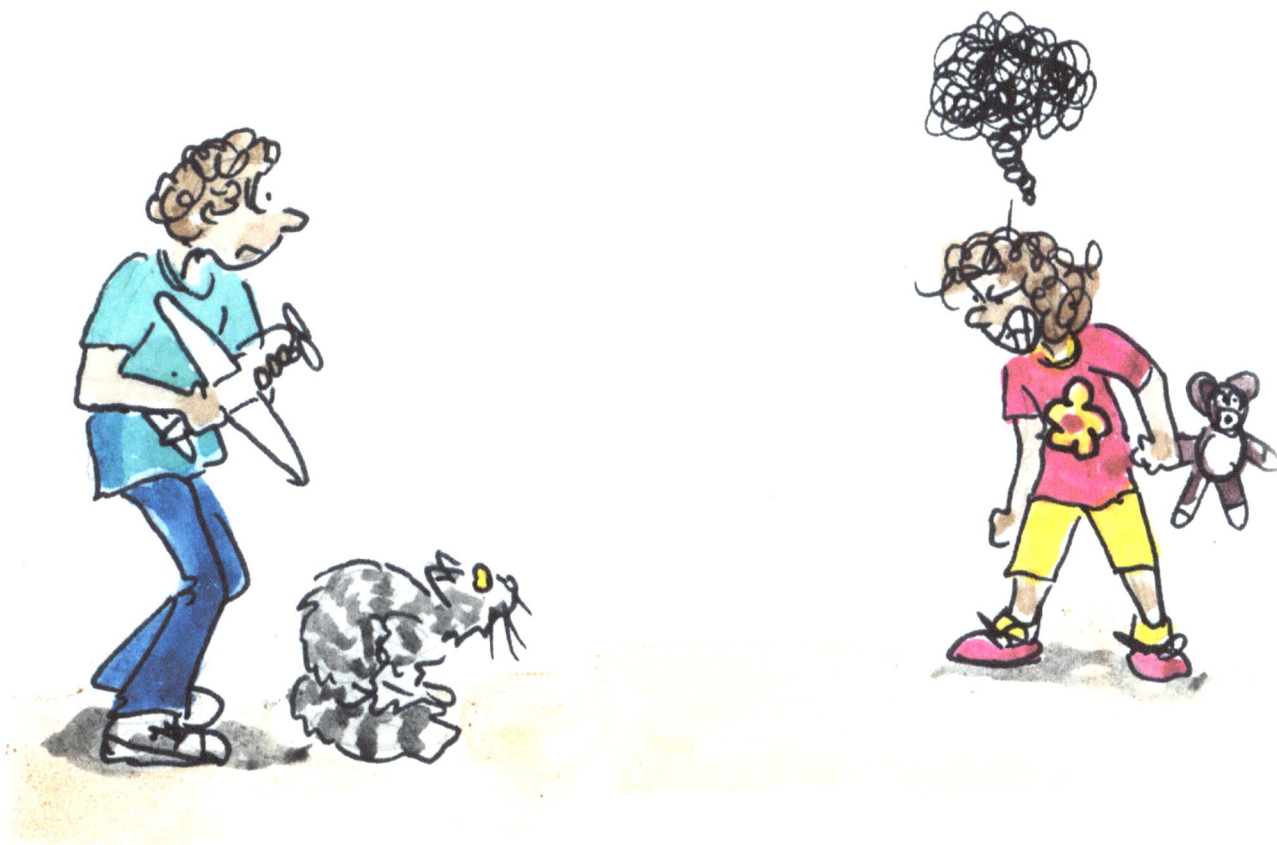

...and that if I slept better "things would be easier around this house!"

I know how to try to be better with my colors

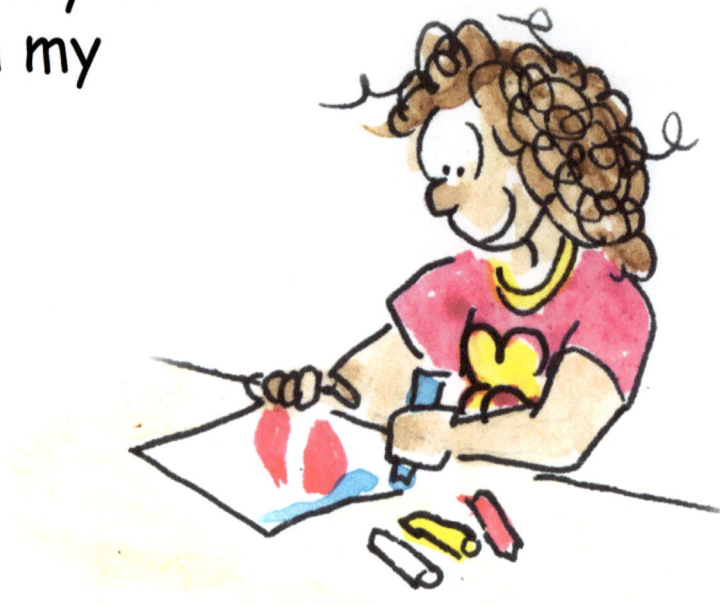

And I practice being better at soccer

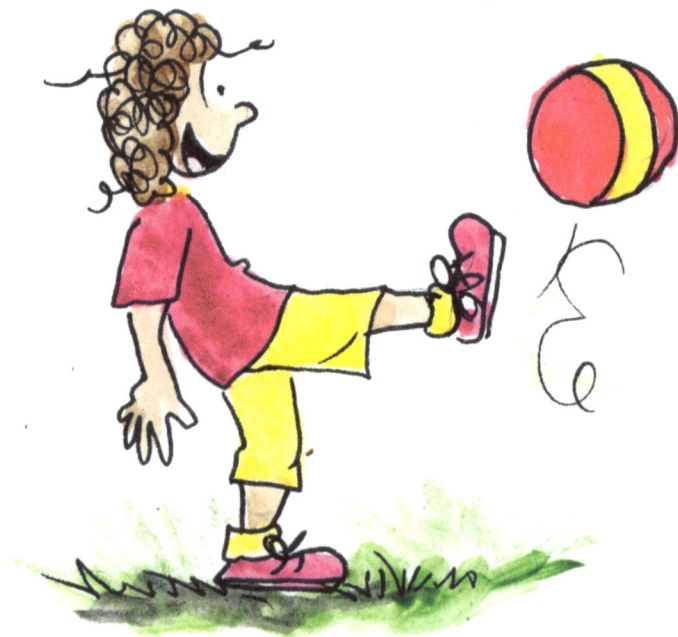

And I try to be
a nice sister

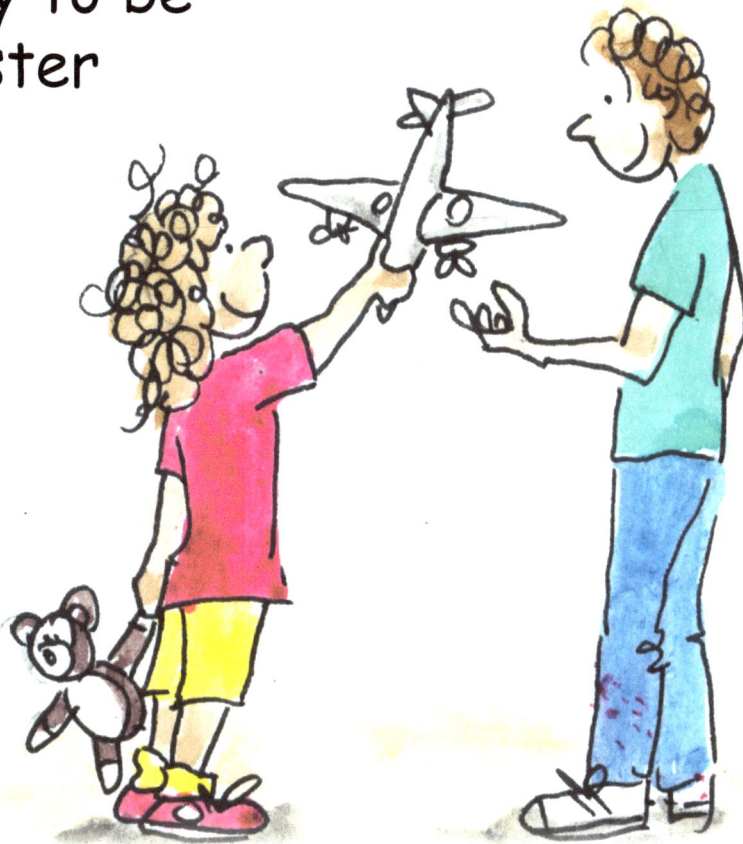

And help around the house, too!

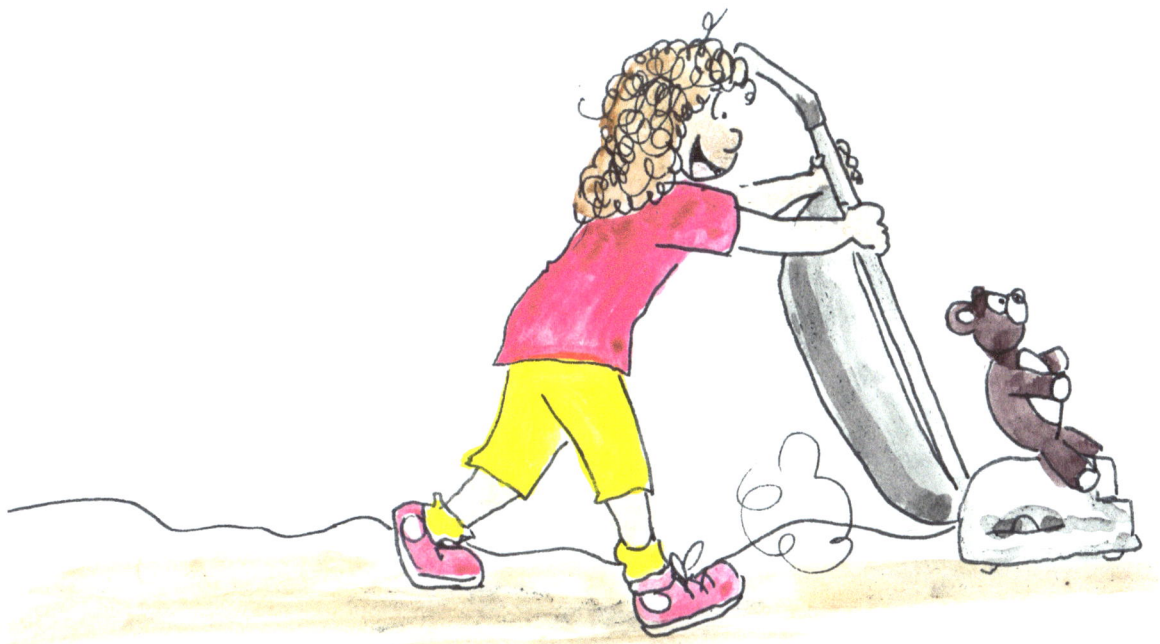

But I don't know how to sleep better...

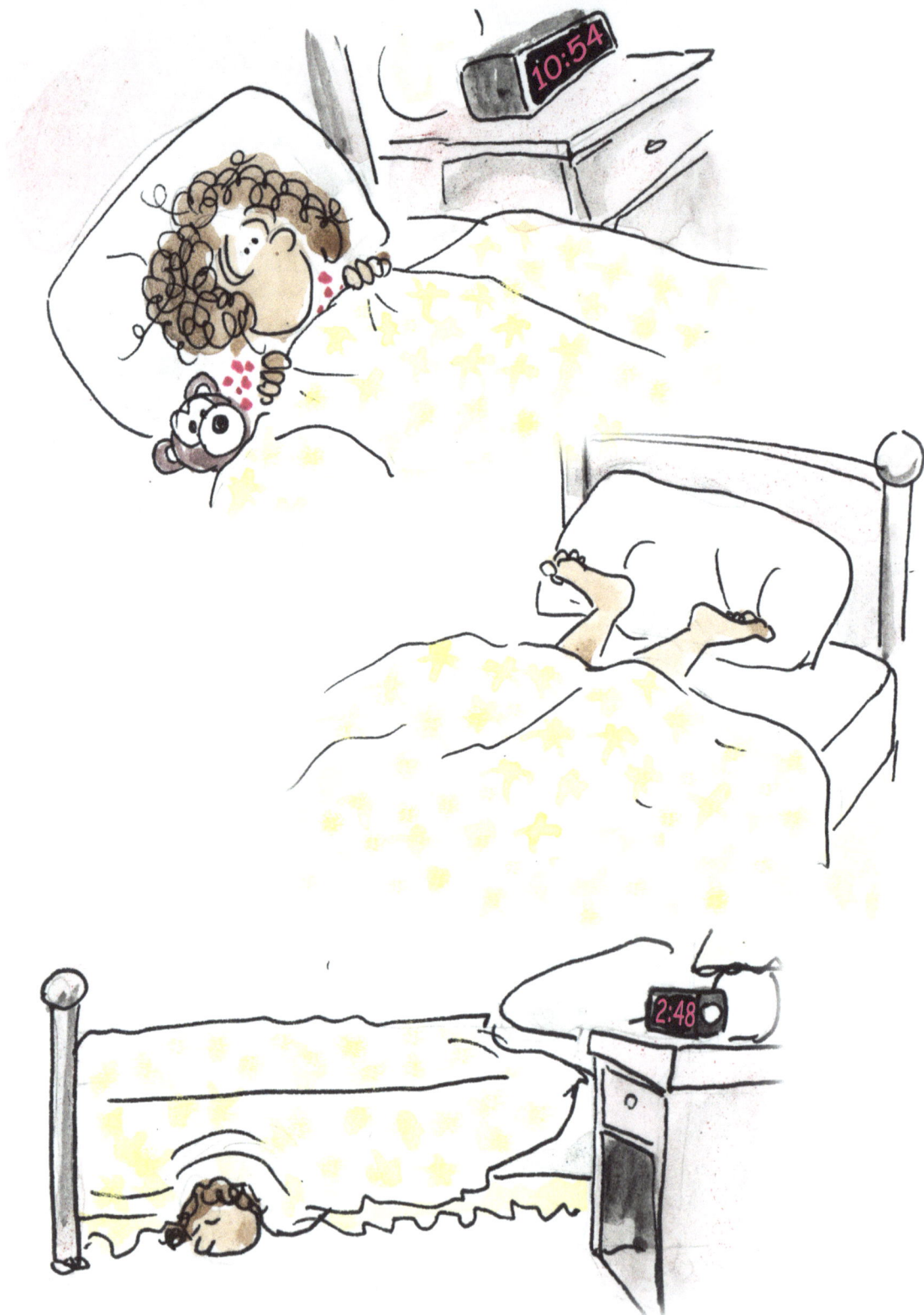

I went to the doctor
and we talked about
my sleeping.

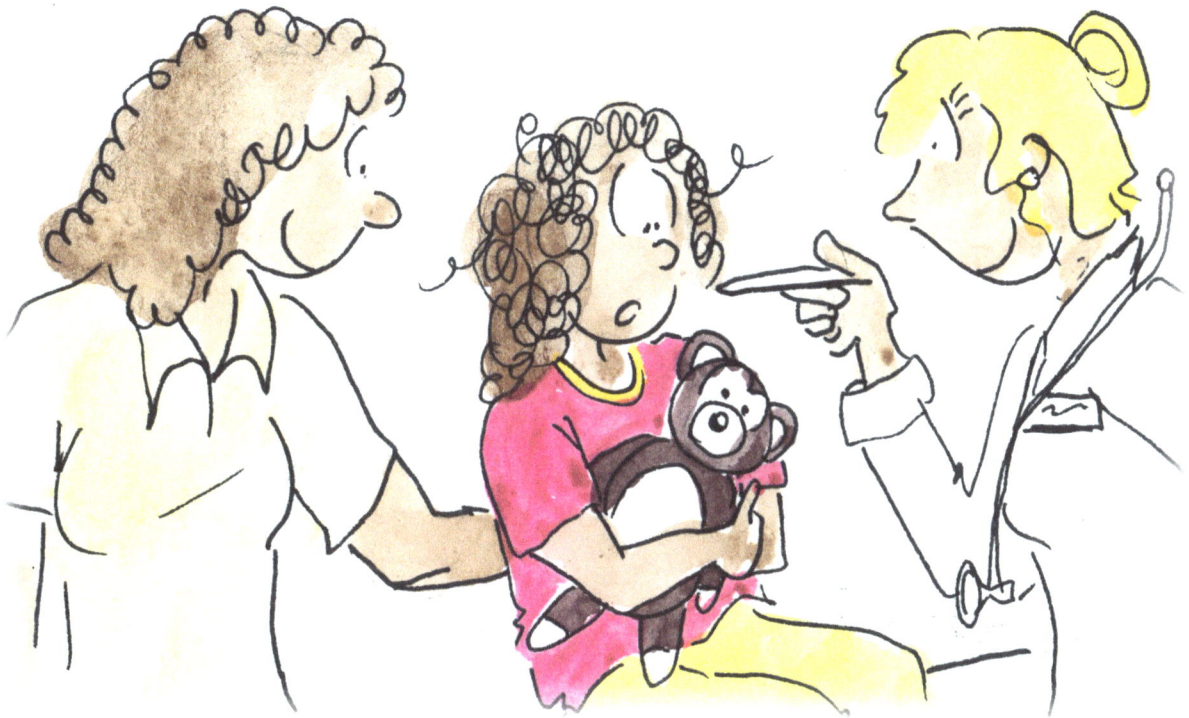

She looked in my throat
and in my ears, and even
in my nose!
YUCK!!

She said I needed to spend the night with some nice people who would watch me sleep. I am sure glad mom went with me!

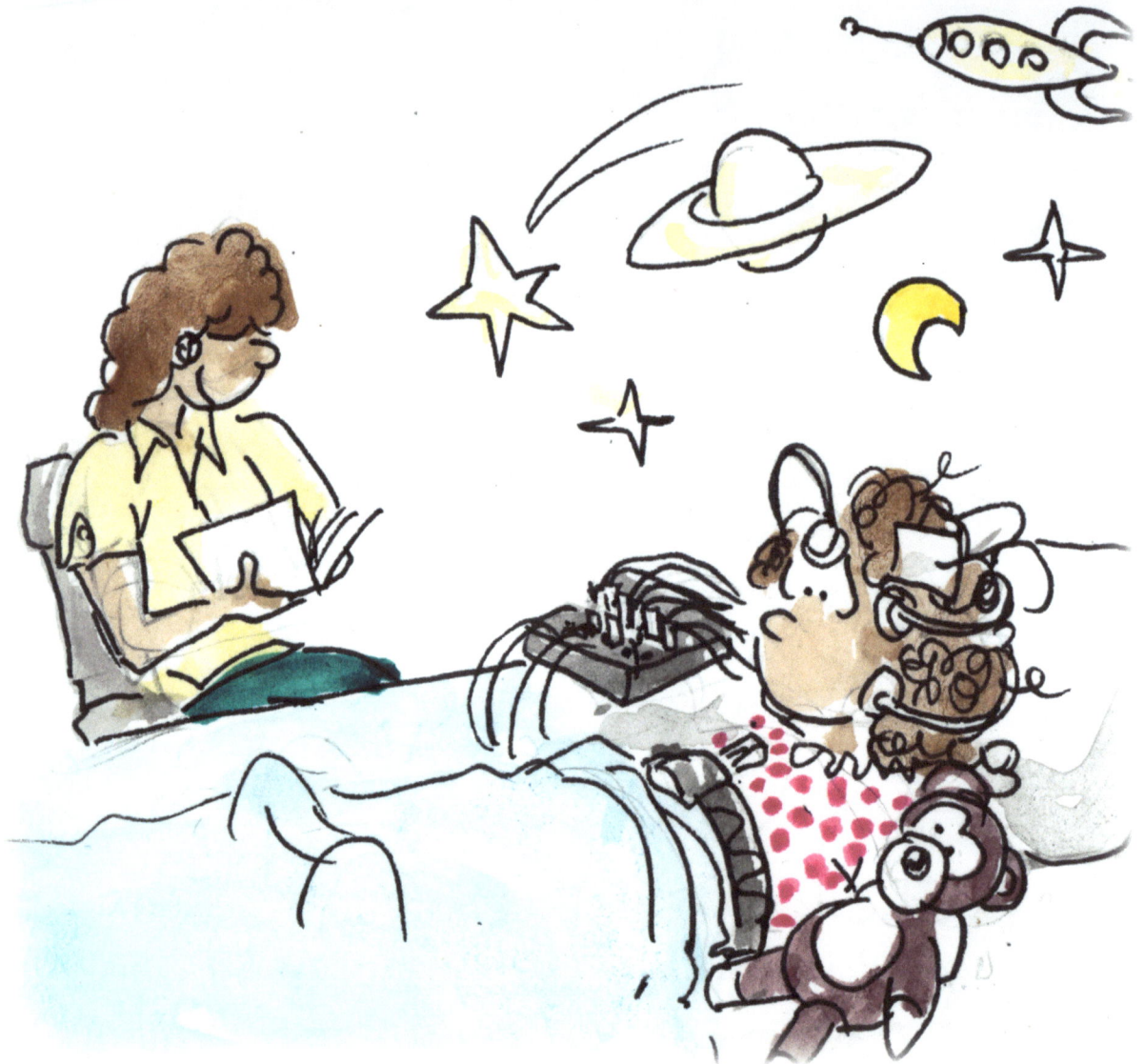

They stuck wires on my head and on my chest! I pretended I was in outer space.

Then I fell asleep.
The people said they
watched me sleep all night
long through a TV.

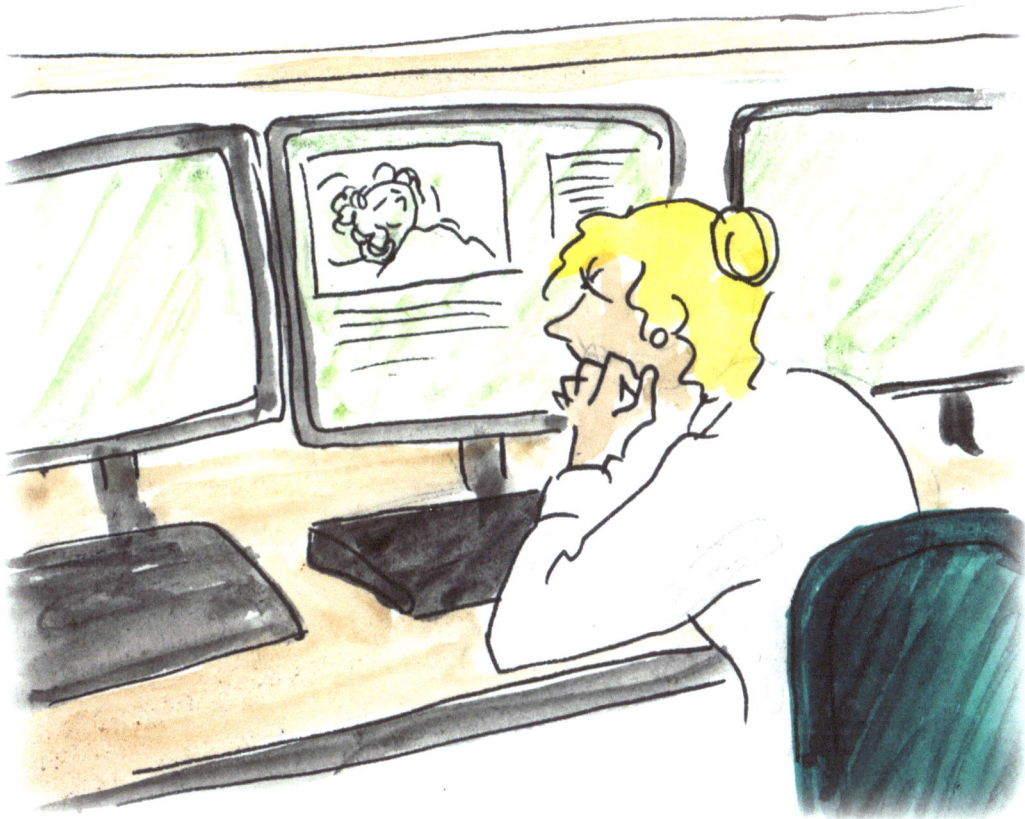

I guess THEY don't sleep very
well either!

In the morning they gave me a machine to help me breathe better so I won't snore.

It is called C PAP.

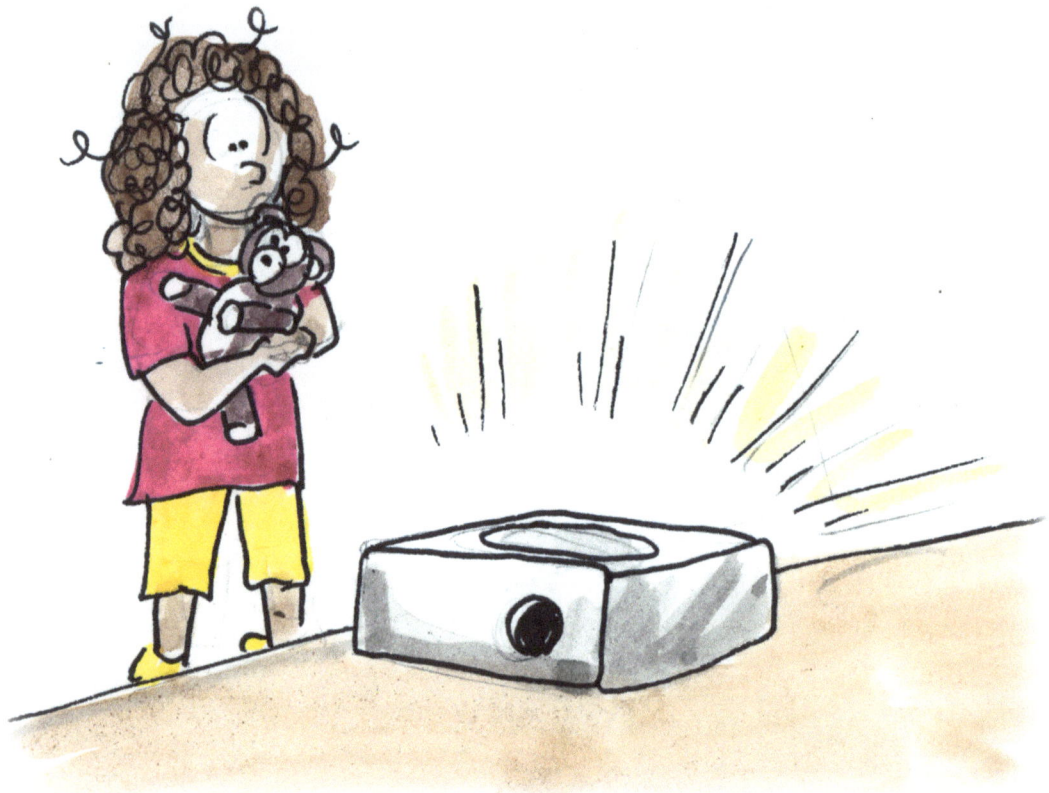

This is one of the words that I can read on my very own.

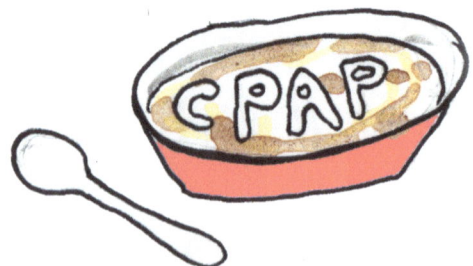

They put a thing on my face they called a mask.

It wasn't like Halloween at all and I was scared at first.

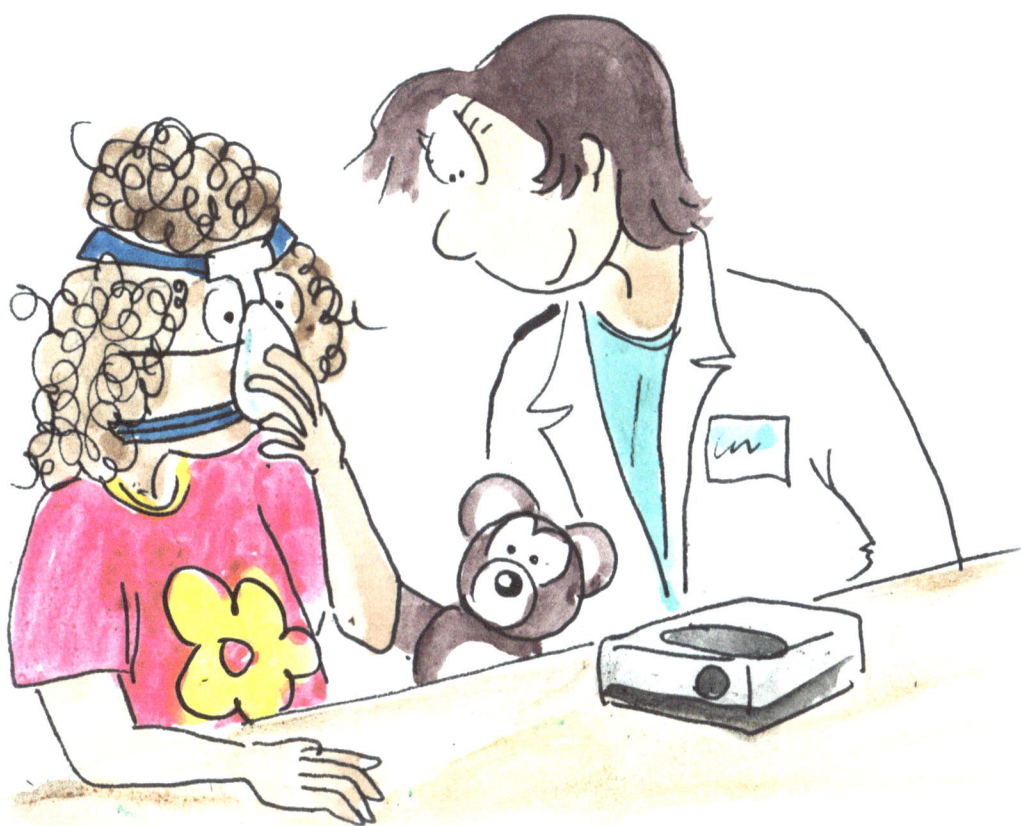

Mom showed me how I could take it off by myself if I had to. She said we would try it again, and it would be OK.

Then we put everything in a bag and took it home.

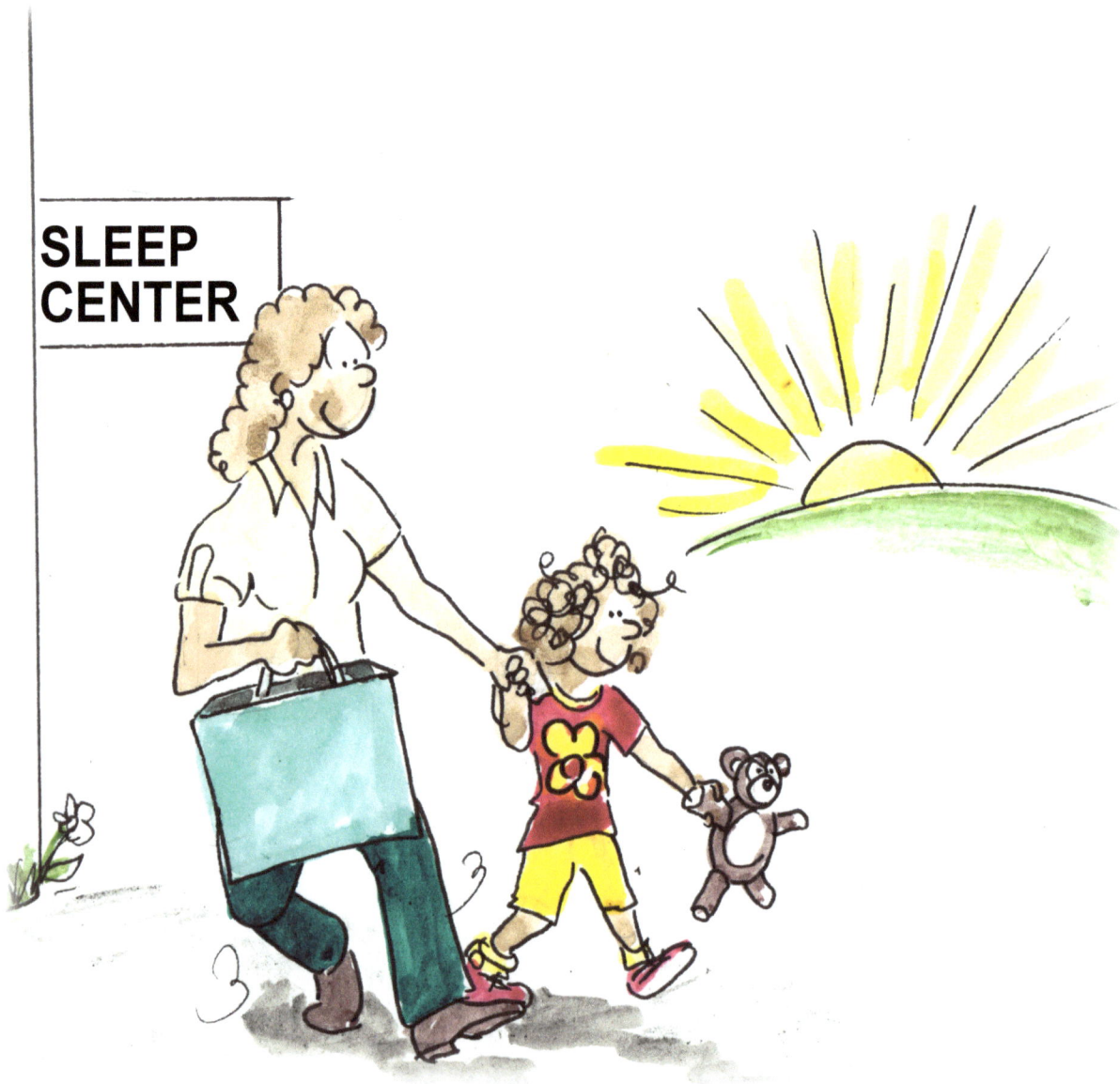

SLEEP
CENTER

I showed it all to my brother. We tried all kinds of things with it.

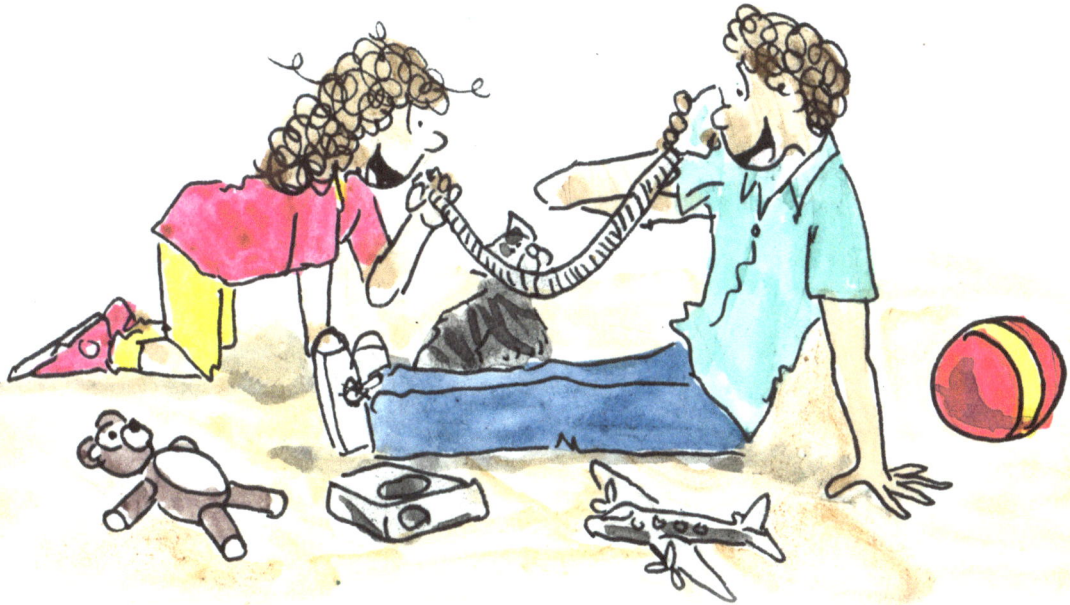

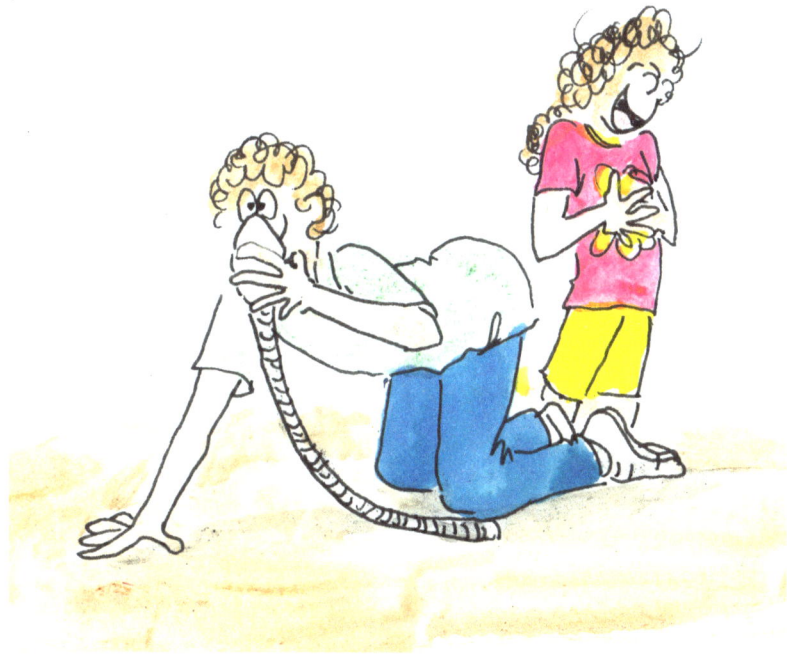

Then we set it up by my bed.

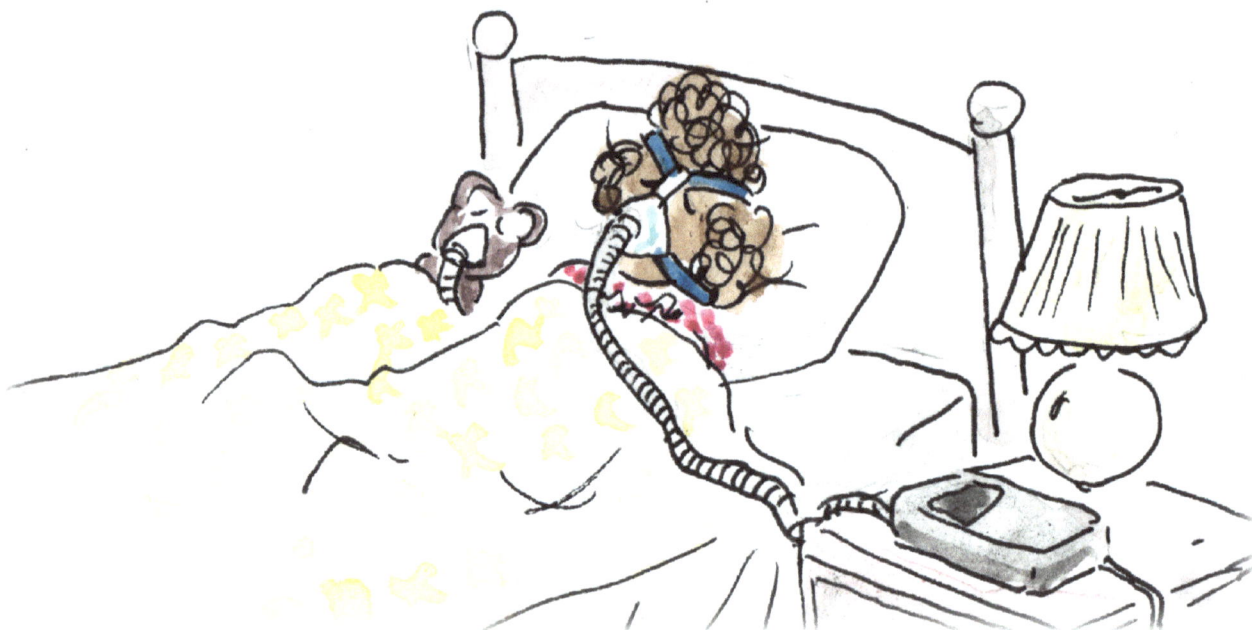

At night I use the machine. It took me a bunch of nights to learn to use it all the time, and now I sleep with it all night long.

My dad says I am not so grumpy now!

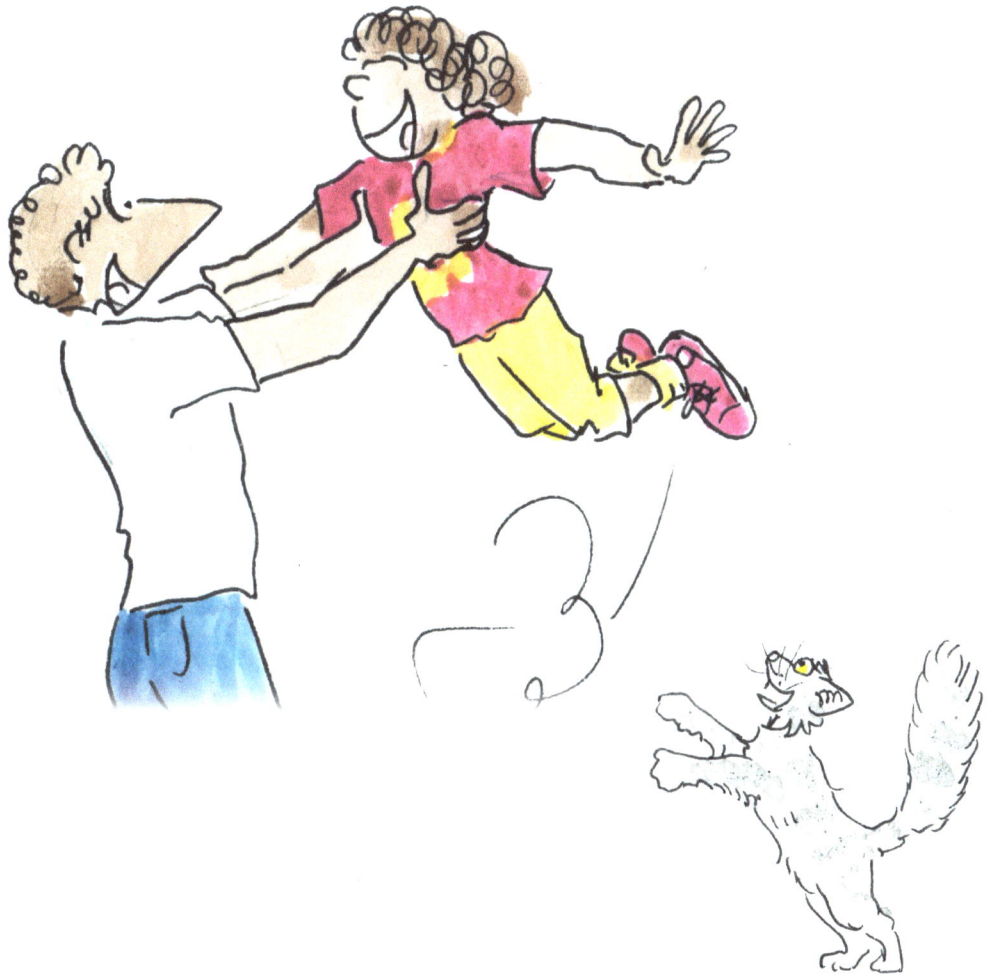

And I don't fall
asleep in school.

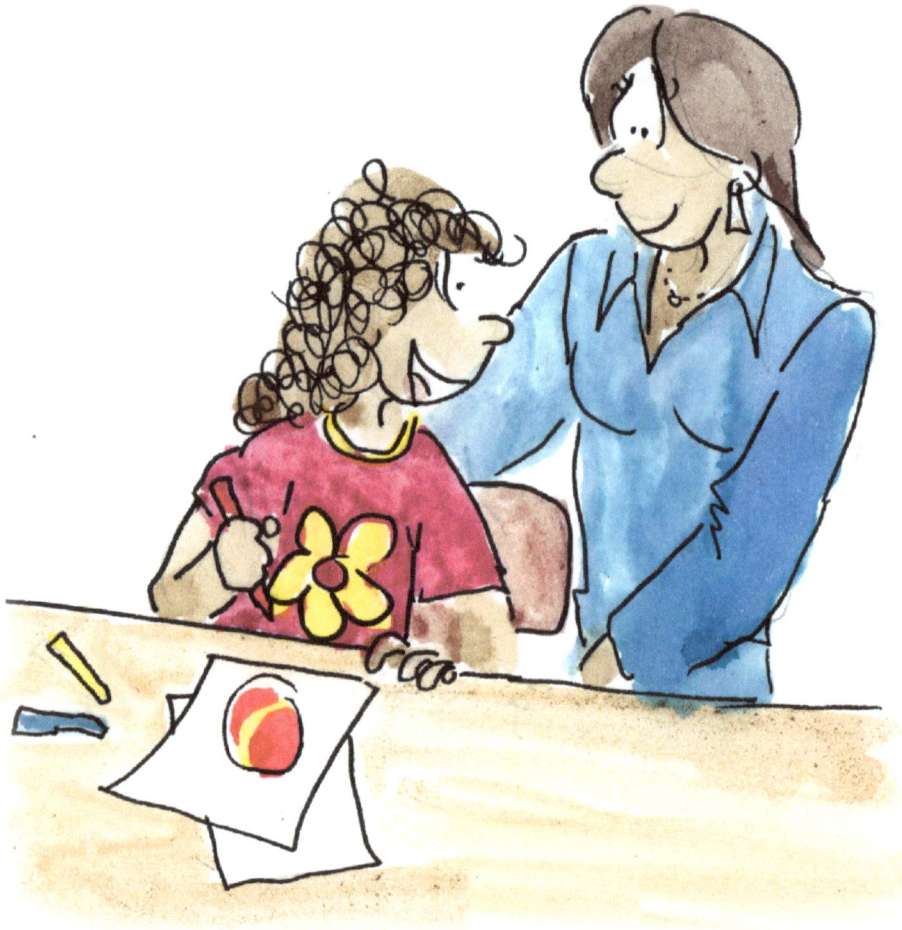

And I get to go to sleep-overs with my friends again. I just take my CPAP with me!

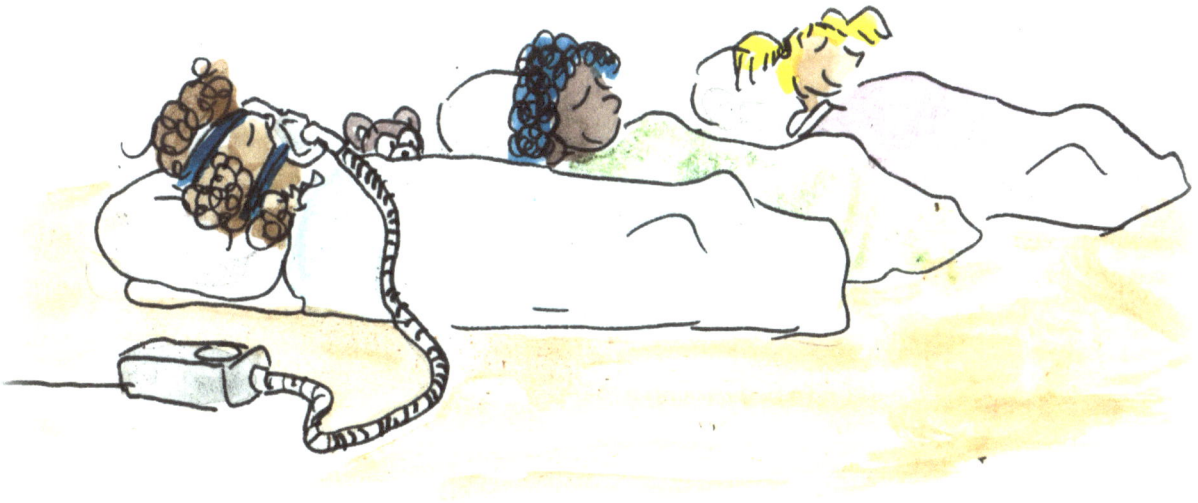

Last week at school we had show-and-tell. I wore my ballerina clothes. A boy named Jamie brought a CPAP!

He showed everyone how he wears it at night.

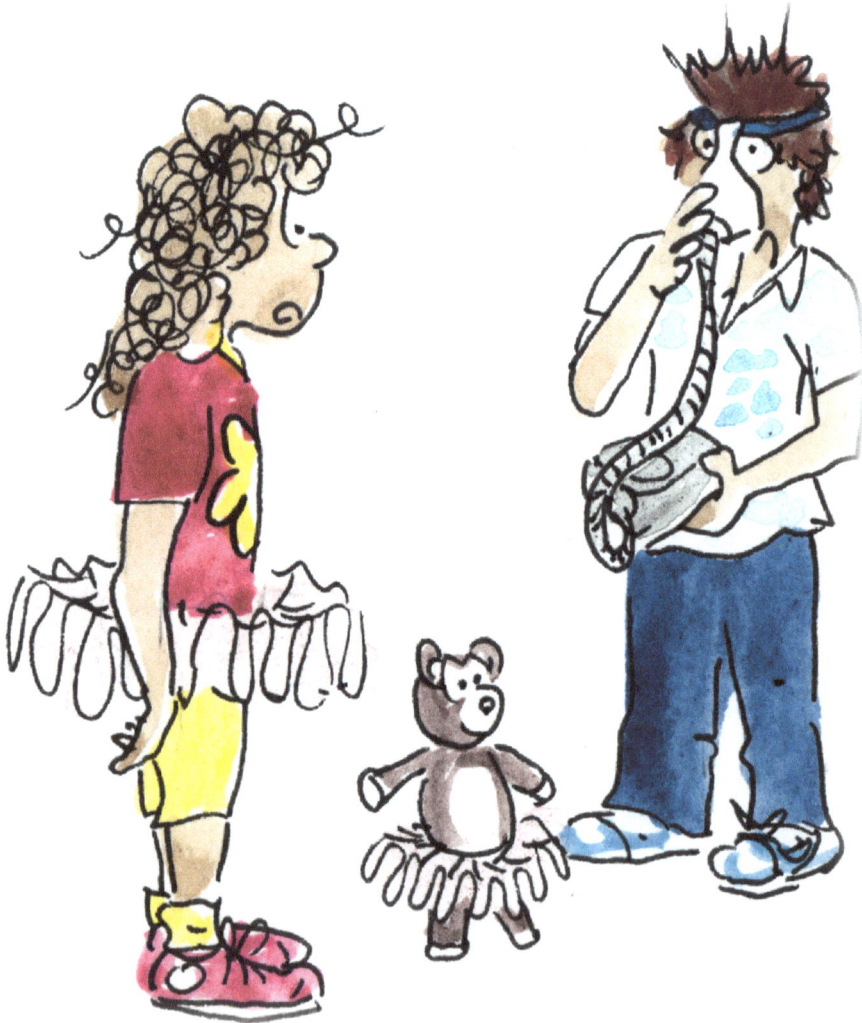

I guess he is extra special too.

I don't think his machine has made him any nicer though.

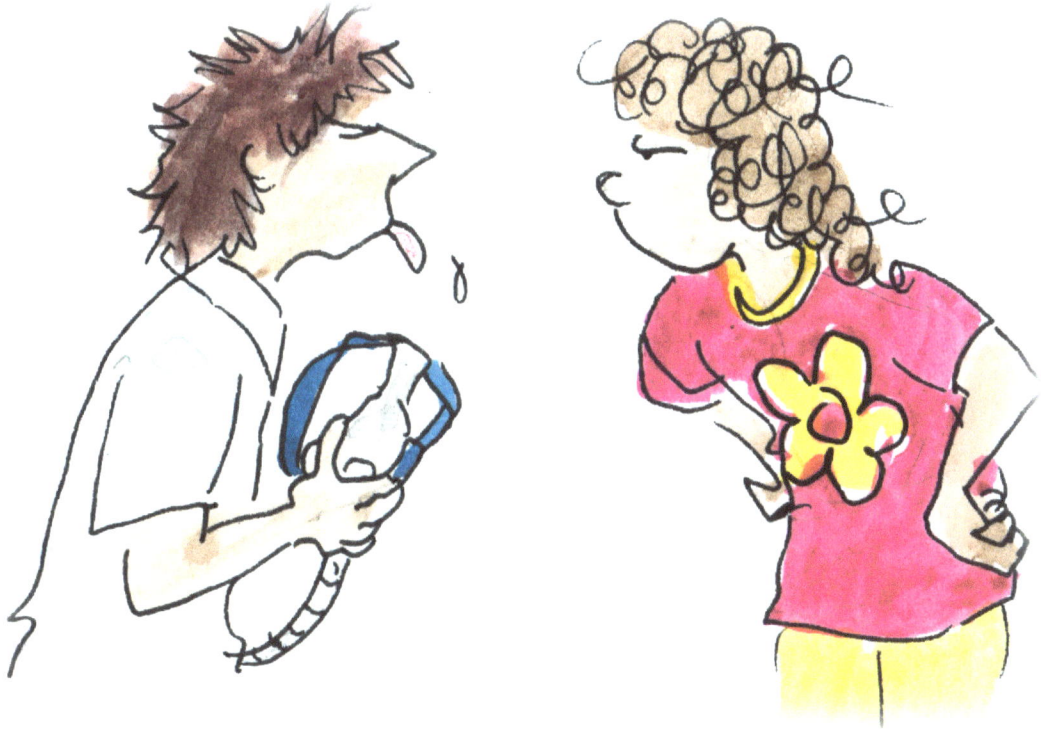

If other kids have trouble sleeping
and they get a CPAP,
I will tell them not to be afraid,
and that...

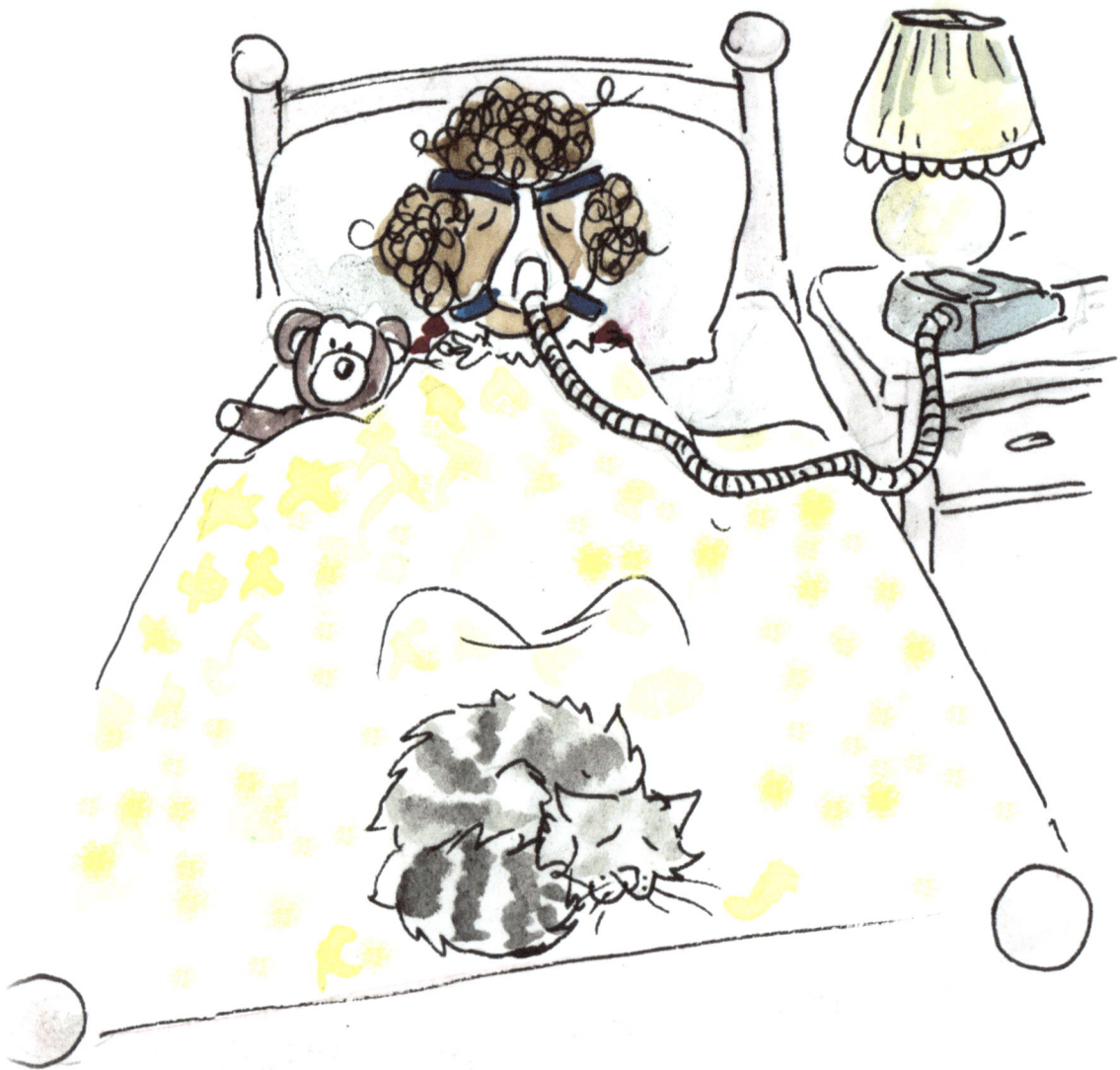

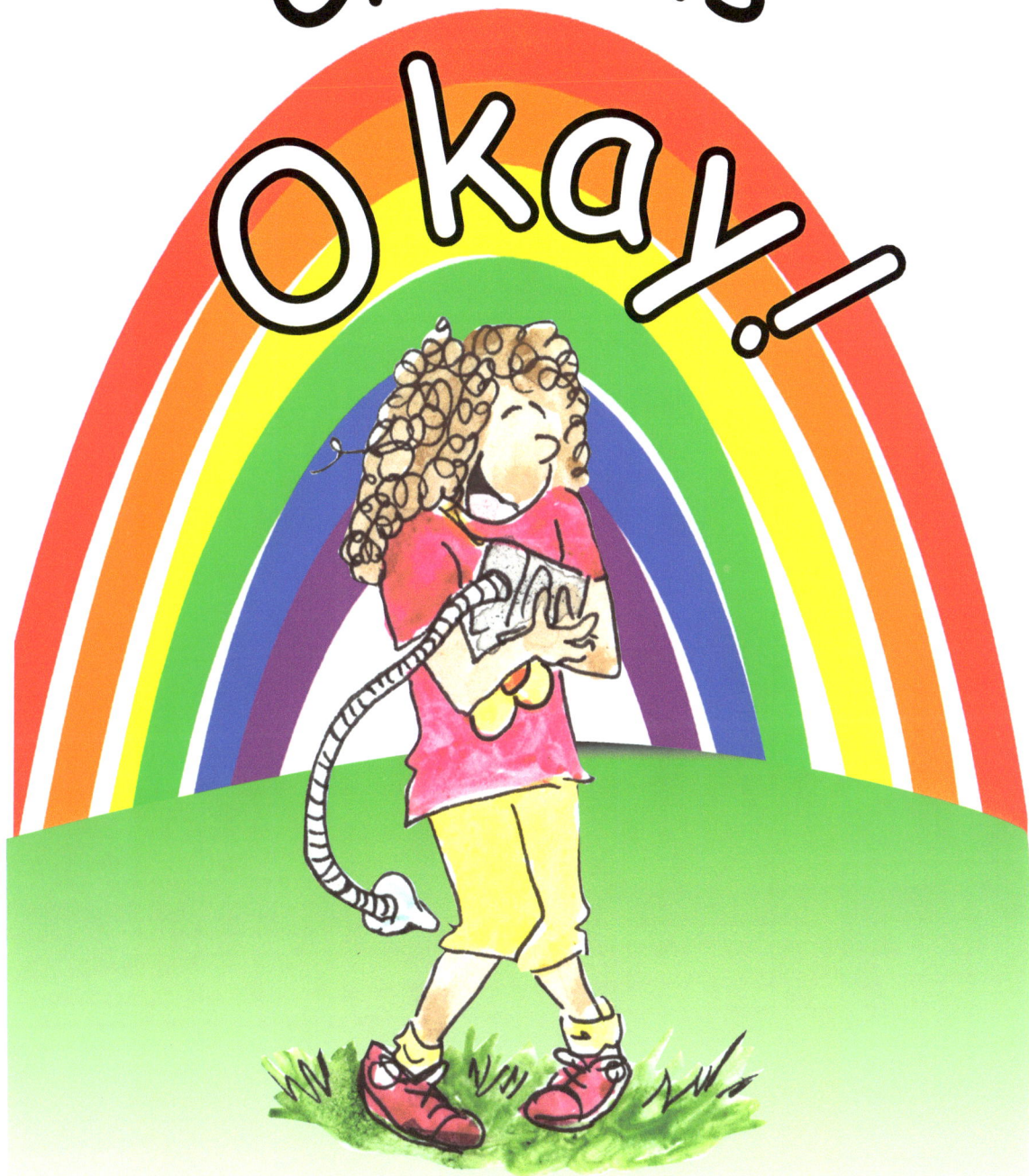
CPAP is Okay!

www.ingramcontent.com/pod-product-compliance
Lightning Source LLC
Chambersburg PA
CBHW052044190326
41520CB00002BA/184